SOCIAL
ANXIETY
DISORDER

POCKET MANUAL

SOCIAL ANXIETY DISORDER

POCKET MANUAL

Jonathan R.T. Davidson, Editor

Director, Anxiety and Traumatic Stress Program
Department of Psychiatry and Behavioral Sciences
Duke University Medical Center
Durham, North Carolina

Brought to you by an unrestricted grant from
SmithKline Beecham Pharmaceuticals

CURRENT MEDICINE, INC.

CURRENT MEDICINE, INC.

© Copyright 1998 by
Current Medicine, Inc.
Philadelphia, Pennsylvania

ISBN: 1-57340-120-X

Development Editor: Lee Tevebaugh
Cover Design: Robert LeBrun
Layout: Patrick Ward
Illustrator: Ann Saydlowski
Production: Lori Holland

Printed in the United States by ANRO

5 4 3 2 1

■ CONTENTS

■ PREFACE

Over the past 5 years, we have learned a great deal about the underlying basis for social anxiety disorder as well as its biologic and psychologic characteristics. Most importantly, we now have in our hands a number of highly effective interventions, which can relieve years of chronic distress and impairment. Of greater priority, however, is the need to teach both health care professionals and the general public that social anxiety disorder is a serious medical disorder, that there is no need for stigma or shame, and that the disorder can be effectively treated. It is in pursuit of these aims that this pocket manual has been written.

Jonathan R.T. Davidson, MD

■ INTRODUCTION

Recently, there has been a dramatic increase in the amount of research conducted in the field of social anxiety disorder, also known as social phobia.

Over the past few years social phobia has progressed from a largely neglected condition to a fully recognized anxiety disorder, acknowledged to cause widespread suffering and disability.

Originally believed to be a relatively rare condition, social anxiety disorder is now estimated to strike at least one in 10 people at some time in their lives.

Sufferers of social anxiety disorder are at considerable risk of comorbidity with conditions such as major depression, agoraphobia, and panic disorder. They have a high rate of alcohol and substance abuse and are almost twice as likely as the general population to attempt suicide.

Much of this impairment and distress could be avoided if the condition were diagnosed earlier and treated more effectively. Unfortunately, social anxiety disorder is underdiagnosed and undertreated. It is believed that between 3% and 25% of social anxiety disorder suffers receive treatment. Most of those who do receive medical help receive inappropriate therapies.

Nevertheless, the diagnostic criteria for social anxiety disorder have, in recent years, become increasingly practical and precise. Advances in treatment have also taken place, allowing physicians to have far greater confidence in their diagnoses of social anxiety disorder. It is now possible to offer real hope of an effective therapy.

This manual is designed to consolidate these research advances into a practical guide to aid practicing physicians in recognizing, diagnosing, and treating social anxiety disorder.

■ EPIDEMIOLOGY

Social anxiety disorder (also known as social phobia) is a widespread and debilitating disorder. Untreated, it is an incapacitating illness that strikes in early adolescence and can continue for the rest of the sufferer's life.

Social phobia does not appear to discriminate greatly between the genders or between social classes. However, because it has detrimental effects on sufferers' education, performance at work, and ability to form relationships, social phobia is diagnosed most often in single people of reduced financial means.

Prevalence

In the early 1960s, when the term *social phobia* was first introduced it was considered to be a relatively rare disorder. However, as diagnostic criteria and interview instruments have become more sophisticated in recent years, social anxiety disorder has been recognized to affect at least one person in 10 at some time in their lives.

Recent European studies have estimated the lifetime prevalence of social anxiety disorder at between 9.6% and 16%. This result is broadly in line with the US estimated lifetime prevalence of 13.3%. Approximately 3% of the US population are suffering social anxiety disorder at any one time.

Age of Onset

Social anxiety disorder tends to strike at a very early age, often during adolescence (*see* Fig. 1). Approximately 40% of social anxiety disorders occur prior to 10 years of age and about 95% before the age of 20 years. This early onset can cause serious development problems.

Education

Most of the large epidemiologic studies have found that sufferers of social anxiety disorder are likely to have a lower level of education than that of healthy control subjects. This outcome has been explained by the detrimental effects of the disorder on sufferers' educational performance.

FIGURE 1

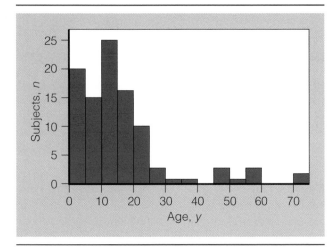

Age at onset of social anxiety disorder. Adapted from Schneier et al., Arch Gen Psychiatry, 1992.

Economic Status

The limitations of social anxiety disorder inevitably have an effect on the financial situation of sufferers. Social anxiety disorder sufferers are, in general, in a lower income bracket than controls and more than 20% are financially dependent on disability or welfare payments.

Cultural Differences

Social anxiety disorder and similar syndromes have been found in almost every culture studied. However, the presentation, recognition, and diagnosis of the condition clearly vary between different societies. Epidemiologic studies suggest that social anxiety disorder is more prevalent in western than eastern societies. This may, however, be due to some cultures regarding fear of social situations as a trait of personality rather than a treatable disorder. The Japanese use the term *Shinka Shitsu* to describe extreme shyness. Many Shinka Shitsu personality types may in fact be suffering social anxiety disorder.

SOCIAL ANXIETY DISORDER AND MARITAL STATUS

Marital status	Social anxiety disorder (n=123)	Without social anxiety disorder (n=3678)
Married, %	47.4	59.4
Widowed, %	7.8	9.8
Divorced, %	11.2	6.0
Separated, %	4.6	3.7
Never married, %	28.7	21.3

From Davidson et al., Psychol Med, 1993.

Marital Status
The detrimental effect of social anxiety disorder on an individual's ability to relate to others is well illustrated by the fact that sufferers of the condition are significantly less likely than healthy control subjects to live with a partner (*see* table).

Gender Distribution
Social anxiety disorder is believed to occur more commonly in women in community-based samples, but in clinical samples the genders are either equally represented or the majority are men.

It may be that men are more likely than women to use coping strategies, such as alcohol. This might lead to an underestimation of male social anxiety disorder in community-based research.

Equally, women might be underrepresented in clinical samples through better opportunities to avoid social phobic situations. A housewife who remains at home all day may never seek treatment and therefore be excluded from the clinical data.

Summary
Social anxiety disorder is a widespread and serious disorder causing significant distress and debilitation throughout several sections of society.

Social anxiety disorder characteristically begins in the mid teenage years—a time when it is likely to cause the greatest damage to psychologic development, the formation of relationships, and the establishment of life goals.

If left unattended, social anxiety disorder may continue to hinder the sufferer's social functioning throughout the rest of his or her life. Sufferers of social anxiety disorder are more likely than healthy control subjects to be living alone, poorly educated, and financially dependent.

■ BURDEN OF SOCIAL ANXIETY DISORDER

If left untreated, social anxiety disorder can lead to a high risk of morbidity, alcoholism, drug abuse, and suicide. These severe consequences inevitably exert a severe burden on individual sufferers, and their friends and family and on society at large.

Personal Burden

Social anxiety disorder is an extremely disabling disorder; it is at least as disabling as panic disorder and is associated with similar impairment to other chronic psychiatric conditions such as depression.

The inability to function in social situations and the tendency to avoid such situations if at all possible have a severe detrimental impact on sufferers' personal, academic, and professional lives.

As many as nine of 10 patients treated for social anxiety disorder claim their condition has had a detrimental effect on their job performance. More than 50% of these patients report using alcohol or benzodiazepines to reduce anxiety in the social situations they forced themselves to attend.

Sufferers of social anxiety disorder are more likely than the general population to

- Be single
- Be less educated
- Be financially dependent
- Be financially less well off
- Suffer additional psychiatric disorders
- Think of suicide
- Commit suicide
- Have an unstable employment record
- Be socially isolated

Alcohol Abuse

According to the World Health Organization, the economic costs of alcohol problems are equivalent to 5% to 6% of the gross national product.

SOCIAL ANXIETY DISORDER IN ALCOHOL ABUSERS

Study	Alcohol abusers, *n*	Social anxiety disorder, %
Chambless *et al.* (1987)	75	21
Strvynski *et al.* (1986)	96	8
Smail *et al.* (1984)	60	39
Bowen *et al.* (1984)	48	8.5
Mullaney and Trippett (1979)	102	56

In 1990, alcohol abuse was estimated to have cost the US economy $120 billion in direct medical costs and indirect costs from crime and loss of productivity. The link between social anxiety disorder and alcohol abuse is therefore of significant economic relevance.

The evidence suggests that patients with social anxiety disorder are more than twice as likely as the general population to have alcohol problems and that people with alcohol problems are nine times as likely to have social anxiety disorder as the general population.

Economic Burden

Social anxiety disorder undoubtedly exerts a heavy economic toll, both on those it immediately effects and on society at large. With its high prevalence and significant degree of associated morbidity, this condition inevitably limits the working and earning potential of large numbers of people.

Although the underrecognition of social anxiety disorder suggests that sufferers are currently not receiving all the health care they require, there is persuasive evidence to suggest that they still account for a considerable amount of health care costs.

The extensive degree of comorbidity in social anxiety disorder means that even if patients are not offered treatment for their social anxiety disorder they are likely to receive it for something else. Social anxiety disorder sufferers have a higher than

DEMOGRAPHIC CHARACTERISTICS

	Social anxiety disorder	Control	Probability
Mean education, y	10.9	11.6	$P=0.01$
Mean income category	7.0	8.2	$P=0.01$
Separated, %	4.6	3.7	$P=0.008$
Employed, %	64.5	63.6	—
Repeatedly fired, %	5.6	1.3	2.00–9.47
Repeatedly absent/late from work, %	16.3	6.4	1.79–4.58

From Davidson et al., Psychol Med, 1993.

average rate of seeking outpatient treatment for emotional problems and of psychiatric outpatient treatment.

Social anxiety disorder sufferers therefore tend to pose a far greater than average burden on health care costs.

Inappropriate treatment also adds to the health care costs of social anxiety disorder. One analysis of treatment offered to social anxiety disorder patients showed that 39% received analytical psychotherapy, for which there is no evidence of efficacy; 82% received supportive counseling; 68% received benzodiazepines, which risk dependency with long-term use; and 32% received tricyclic antidepressants, which, based on current knowledge, are probably not effective. Cognitive therapy and monoamine oxidase inhibitors (MAOIs), both of which have shown efficacy in trials, were offered to only 4% of the patients.

Burden on Young People

With its early onset and provocation of fear under scrutiny or when being judged, social anxiety disorder is a particularly damaging disorder for school children. School is an inherently social situation and, as might be expected, children with social anxiety disorder are prone to a much higher than average degree of educational difficulties. Some 43% have anxiety-based school refusal. Examination of school refusers shows that at least 30% are suffering from social anxiety disorder.

USE OF MEDICAL SERVICES IN SOCIAL ANXIETY DISORDER (RATE/100)

Treatment sought	Uncomplicated (n = 112)	Comorbid (n = 249)	No disorder (n = 9953)
Any outpatient	19.6	51.0	14.7
Medical outpatient	17.0	28.9	9.2
Psychiatric outpatient	5.4	37.8	7.9
Emergency department	1.8	11.2	1.4
Psychiatric inpatient	0.9	13.7	1.5

From Schneier et al., Arch Gen Psychiatry, 1992.

The result is that school performance is seriously impaired and long-term consequences are almost inevitable. Children with social anxiety disorder grow into adults who are at higher than average risk of social impairment, employment difficulties, and further psychiatric illness.

Early onset of social anxiety disorder is a particularly serious problem because of the effect of the illness at a vulnerable age when social coping skills are being developed. If a child never learns the mechanisms of social interaction the effects can restrict his or her adult life.

Nonrecognition of Social Anxiety Disorder
Two studies have shown that physicians fail to recognize the vast majority of cases of social anxiety disorder. In one US community survey, only 3% of patients suffering from social anxiety disorder had received treatment in the past year. The physician recognition rate was only 10% in cases in which a psychologic problem was detected. In a general practice study, the current prevalence of social anxiety disorder was 4.9%. Less than one half of nondepressed patients with social anxiety disorder were noted to have any type of psychologic problem by the doctor.

Summary

Social anxiety disorder is a debilitating, chronic, largely unremitting disorder, which, if left untreated, can lead to a high risk of morbidity, alcoholism, drug abuse, and suicide.

The personal and financial costs of the condition are extremely high. Sufferers are restricted in their social life, education, and professional activities. These restrictions significantly impair their quality of life, earning potential, and contribution to society at large.

Direct costs to the health service include a higher than average consultation rate for a wide range of comorbid disorders.

Earlier recognition and treatment of social anxiety disorder could avoid considerable personal impairment and distress and help reduce a significant financial burden.

■ PRESENTATION AND DIAGNOSIS

The essential features of social anxiety disorder are

- Fear of scrutiny by other people in social situations
- Marked and persistent fear of performance situations in which embarrassment or humiliation may occur
- Avoidance of the feared situations

Individuals with social anxiety disorder have a disproportionate fear of being negatively evaluated in a wide range of social situations.

The condition may be generalized, in which the fears involve almost all social contacts, or nongeneralized, in which the fears relate to specific social activities or performance situations.

The most common precipitating situations include

- Being introduced
- Meeting people in authority
- Using the telephone
- Receiving visitors
- Being watched doing something
- Being teased
- Eating at home with acquaintances
- Eating at home with family
- Writing in front of others
- Speaking in public

When exposed to the feared situation, sufferers of social anxiety disorder frequently experience somatic symptoms of anxiety such as palpitations, trembling, sweating, tense muscles, a sinking feeling in the stomach, dry throat, hot or cold feelings, or headache.

The sufferer may be convinced that one of the secondary manifestations of anxiety is the primary problem. Some sufferers, however, do not complain of somatic symptoms but experience great self-consciousness, fear, and apprehension.

Avoidance of the feared situations is often marked and in extreme cases may lead to almost complete social isolation.

Attempted suicide and suicidal ideation are common in social anxiety disorder. A sufferer with the comorbid condition is more than five times more likely than the general population to make an attempt on his or her own life. The risk of suicide ideation in comorbid social anxiety disorder is higher than in comorbid panic disorder.

Diagnostic Criteria for Social Anxiety Disorder (DSM-IV)

1. A marked and persistent fear of one or more social performance situations in which the person is exposed to unfamiliar people or to possible scrutiny by other. The individual fears that he or she will act in a way (or show anxiety symptoms) that will be humiliating or embarrassing. **Note:** In children, there must be evidence of the capacity for age-appropriate social relationships with familiar people and the anxiety must occur in peer settings, not just in interactions with adults.

2. Exposure to the feared social situation almost invariably provokes anxiety, which may take the form of a situationally bound or situationally predisposed panic attack. **Note:** In children, the anxiety may be expressed by crying, throwing tantrums, freezing, or shrinking from social situations with unfamiliar people.

3. The person recognizes that the fear is excessive or unreasonable. **Note:** In children, this feature may be absent.

4. The feared social or performance situations are avoided or else are endured with intense anxiety or distress.

5. The avoidance, anxious anticipation, or distress in the feared social or performance situation interferes significantly with the person's normal routine, occupational or academic functioning, or social activities or relationships, or there is marked distress about having the phobia.

6. In individuals less than 18 years of age, the duration is at least 6 months.

7. The fear or avoidance is not due to the direct physiologic effects of a substance (*eg*, drug of abuse, medication) of a general medical condition and is not better accounted for by another mental disorder (*eg*, panic disorder with or without agoraphobia, separation anxiety disorder, body dysmorphic disorder, a pervasive developmental disorder, or schizoid personality disorder).

8. If a general medical condition or another mental disorder is present, the fear in criterion 1 is unrelated to it, *eg*, the fear is not of stuttering, trembling in Parkinson's disease, or exhibiting abnormal eating behavior in anorexia nervosa or bulimia nervosa.

Specify if:

Generalized—the fears include most social situations (also consider the additional diagnosis of avoidant personality disorder).

Differences Between DSM-IV and ICD-10

There is broad agreement between ICD-10 and DSM-IV as to what constitutes social anxiety disorder. Essential differences include

- Panic disorder
  In DSM-IV panic disorder takes precedence over social anxiety disorder if both are present, whereas ICD-10 stipulates that panic disorder "should be diagnosed only in the absence of any of the other phobic disorders' including social anxiety disorder."

- Agoraphobia
  ICD-10 suggests that if the distinction between social anxiety disorder and agoraphobia is very difficult, precedence should be given to agoraphobia. DSM-IV differentiates between the two conditions on the basis of the fear of scrutiny.

Decision Trees

It has been estimated that only 3% to 25% of social anxiety disorder sufferers ever receive treatment. Most of those who do receive medical help receive inappropriate therapies. There are several reasons why the condition may go unrecognized, including the presence of comorbid conditions and the perception among patients and medical profession that the symptoms are traits of personality rather than signs of a treatable illness. The decision tree may help to improve the recognition of patients with social anxiety disorder (*see* Fig. 2).

Differential Diagnosis

The diagnosis of social anxiety disorder is often complicated by the fact that sufferers may present complaining of secondary features of anxiety, which they interpret as the primary problem. However, careful questioning can clarify whether the situations in which such symptoms occur are generalized or specifically social.

Agoraphobia with or without panic disorder

- Social anxiety disorder is characterized by social fear–avoidance in agoraphobia is based primarily on the fear of having a panic attack or losing control in social situations from which easy escape and exit are difficult or impossible.

- In social anxiety disorder the key element is the fear of being scrutinized–in agoraphobia the feared situations are more generalized.

- In ICD-10, social anxiety disorder takes precedence over panic disorder, but in DSM-IV panic disorder comes first.

- By taking a careful clinical history the physician can distinguish social anxiety disorder by pinpointing the core clinical feature–the fear of scrutiny and humiliation in social situations.

Extreme shyness

- The diagnosis of social anxiety disorder depends on being able to identify some degree of social or occupational impairment.

- Shyness tends to be generalized rather than focused on particular activities.

FIGURE 2

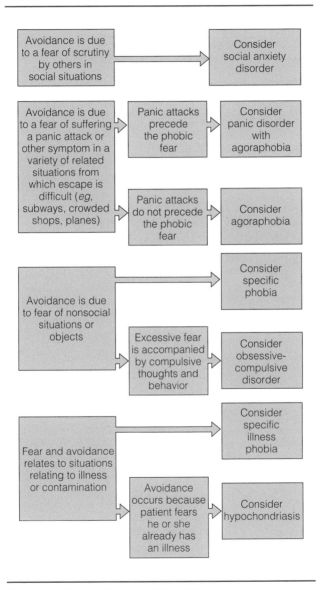

Decision tree used by a patient experiencing phobic avoidance.

Depression

- Social anxiety disorder sufferers withdraw from public situations. Due to the fear of scrutiny, depression may cause individuals to withdraw from social situations, but this is because of a lack of enjoyment.

Alcoholism

- In most cases the social anxiety disorder precedes the alcohol intake and the length of time taken from the development of social anxiety disorder to using alcohol as a prop normally helps distinguish the two conditions.

Social anxiety secondary to another condition

- Individuals with conditions such as Parkinson's disease or stuttering may suffer embarrassment in social situations. At present these social phobic symptoms are not considered as social anxiety disorder.

A Case Study

Mr. LT, a married man aged 39 years was referred by his physician for evaluation and treatment of anxiety. His panic attacks started at the age of 21, worsening over the year prior to coming in for assessment. He was having at least one major panic attack per week, characterized by symptoms of dizziness, chest pain, hot and cold flushes, feelings of apprehension and feelings that the world was going to end. These attacks occurred only during specific social situations such as when he had to give a speech at work. He had also developed phobia to the point at which he refused to attend social events, because he was afraid of embarrassing himself when he spoke. Secondary depressive symptoms included sadness, hopelessness about his panic attacks, and mild hypochondriac tendencies.

A review of Mr. LT's history showed that he had school phobia and was always afraid to get up in front of the class to make presentations. These symptoms occurred many years before the onset of the panic attacks and were always present as he grew up. In his job he was unable to chair meetings and refused promotions because of this.

One of Mr. LT's brothers had also suffered panic attacks, and he described his other siblings as intense and obsessive. His mother had a major depression but was never treated.

Medically he was physically well with exemplary personal habits. He did not smoke cigarettes, drink alcohol, or use illicit drugs. He even avoided caffeine.

On the self-rated Social Anxiety Symptom Scale (*see* Appendix A), Mr. LT rated his symptom at a total score of 42, which is substantially higher than the threshold score of 19, which distinguishes between those individuals with and those without social anxiety disorder.

Mental status showed anxiety and some mild symptoms of depression but no other psychiatric illness.

Assessment
It is quite clear from the patient's history that he developed the social anxiety disorder symptoms prior to the panic attacks. He has a fear of a number of social situations and avoids occasions that involve social interaction.

This behavior started when he was in school and continued throughout his adult life.

The panic attacks that developed as he grew older occurred in social or performance situations. His avoidance behavior limits his professional and financial success because he is refusing promotions that would require more public speaking and social interaction.

The panic attacks do not meet the criteria for panic disorder in DSM-IV because they are related to social or performance situations. The phobia and depressive symptoms developed after the panic attacks began. Although the depressive symptoms are troubling, he does not meet the criteria for depressive disorder.

DSM-IV diagnosis
Social anxiety disorder.

Summary

Social anxiety disorder is centered around a fear of scrutiny by other people in small or large groups or by individual authority figures.

- This fear may be discrete:
  Eating in public
  Public speaking
  Encounters with the opposite sex
- Or diffuse:
  Almost all social situations outside the family circle

When exposed to the feared situations, sufferers frequently experience somatic symptoms of anxiety. The sufferer may be convinced that one of the secondary manifestations of anxiety is the primary problem. Some sufferers, however, do not complain of somatic symptoms but experience great self-consciousness, fear, and apprehension.

Differential diagnoses with agoraphobia should focus on the patient's source of fear.

In social anxiety disorder the primary fear is of scrutiny and humiliation in social situations, whereas agoraphobics primarily fear having a panic attack or losing control in situations from which they cannot escape.

In depression a patient may withdraw from social contact through lack of enjoyment. This is in contrast to a social phobic who withdraws through fear of the scrutiny involved in social contact.

Alcoholics can be distinguished from social phobics who drink to cope with their condition by considering the length of time taken from the development of social anxiety disorder to using alcohol as a prop.

It is important not to dismiss social anxiety disorder as mere shyness but to register the degree of disability. Although many features of social anxiety disorder are common, this does not mean they are trivial. Social phobics suffer considerable interference with their lives and marked distress.

■ COMORBID CONDITIONS

Comorbidity in social anxiety disorder is extremely common. Less than one third of social anxiety disorder sufferers will experience no other psychiatric disorders in their lifetime.

In most cases, the symptoms of social anxiety disorder precede those of the comorbid disorder, suggesting that the presence of social anxiety disorder precipitates the onset of the comorbidity.

Social anxiety disorder has been found to be the primary disorder in 70.9% of the people with comorbid depression, 76.7% of those with comorbid drug abuse, and 85% of those with comorbid alcohol abuse.

The earlier detection and treatment of social anxiety disorder could therefore help prevent the onset of the secondary conditions.

Prevailing Comorbid Conditions

The most frequent comorbid disorders affecting social phobics in the community are

- Simple phobia (59%)
- Agoraphobia (44.9%)
- Alcohol abuse (19%)
- Major depression (17%)
- Drug abuse (17%)

There is also an association between social anxiety disorder and the subsequent onset of eating disorders.

Significance of Comorbidity

If simple, uncomplicated social anxiety disorder is a distressing and debilitating condition, the comorbid condition is undoubtedly worse. Comorbid social phobics appear to suffer a much higher degree of distress and are at far greater risk of the condition's more serious consequences.

For instance, comorbid social anxiety disorder is far more likely to lead to suicide than is the uncomplicated condition.

LIFETIME RISKS OF COMORBID CONDITIONS IN SOCIAL ANXIETY DISORDER

	Social anxiety disorder, % (*n* = 123)	Nonsocial anxiety disorder, % (*n* = 3678)
Psychiatric disorders		
Schizophrenia/schizophreniform	13.3	1.1
Simple phobia	60.8	15.6
Agoraphobia	45.0	6.3
Generalized anxiety	26.9	8.0
Obsessive-compulsive disorder	18.6	2.6
Panic disorder	11.6	1.2
Posttraumatic stress disorder	5.4	0.6
Mania	1.5	0.2
Major depression	14.6	3.4
Alcohol abuse/dependency	17.2	8.3
Suicide		
Attempted suicide	12.1	1.0
Mental disorders		
Neurologic disorder	1.9	0.5
Peptic ulcer disease	9.0	4.7

From Davidson et al., Psychol Med, 1993.

Patients with comorbid social anxiety disorder are 5.73 times more likely than the general population to make an attempt on their own life. Suicidal ideation in comorbid social anxiety disorder is about the same as in comorbid panic disorder (34% vs 31%).

Even though most studies have found that the onset of social anxiety disorder predates the development of any comorbidity, patients are more likely to receive medical treatment for the secondary condition.

In only 11.5% of patients with social anxiety disorder who receive treatment is the therapy specifically aimed at phobia. Social anxiety disorder sufferers are far more likely to receive

SUICIDALITY IN SIMPLE AND COMORBID SOCIAL ANXIETY DISORDER

	Data from ECA studies	
	Simple, %	Comorbid, %
Suicide attempts	0.9	15.7
Thought a lot about death	26.8	53.8
Felt like you wanted to die	8.9	27.7
Felt so low you wanted to commit suicide	9.8	37.3

From Schneier et al, Arch Gen Psychiatry, 1992.

therapy for other forms of anxiety (34.6%), depression (42.3%), or panic disorder (19.2%).

Summary

Far from being the exception, it appears that comorbidity is the rule for patients with social anxiety disorder. Indeed, the diagnosis of uncomplicated, noncomorbid social anxiety disorder almost certainly indicates the need to probe for the existence of other psychiatric disorders.

When social anxiety disorder appears in association with another disorder, it is important not to allow one condition to take precedence over the other.

A wide range of comorbid conditions have been described for social anxiety disorder. These include

- Agoraphobia
- Obsessive-compulsive disorder
- Panic disorder
- Major depression
- Alcohol abuse/dependency
- Eating disorders
- Posttraumatic stress disorder

The finding that social anxiety disorder appears to be the primary disorder in most cases of comorbidity suggests it could precipitate the onset of the subsequent condition. The earlier detection and treatment of simple social anxiety disorder could therefore help prevent comorbidity and thereby save many patients from a great deal of disability and distress.

Patients who suffer comorbid social anxiety disorder face significantly greater disability than those with the uncomplicated condition and are more likely to attempt suicide.

■ TREATMENT OF SOCIAL ANXIETY DISORDER

Introduction

The severe impairment, development of harmful coping strategies and the onset of comorbid conditions associated with the condition can all be prevented or alleviated by early administration of pharmacologic and/or psychologic therapies. It is therefore crucial that once the diagnosis of social anxiety disorder is made, effective treatment strategies are introduced without delay.

Unfortunately only very few sufferers currently receive any therapy at all and substantially fewer receive treatment of proven efficacy.

When to treat

Social anxiety disorder should be treated whenever it causes personal distress, when adequate or optimal function is not being attained due to symptoms, or when avoidance is marked. With the availability of simple, well-tolerated treatments that carry a high rate of success, it is becoming increasingly important to treat social anxiety disorder as early as possible, rather than waiting until it becomes more severe. However, even severe and disabling forms of the disorder respond well to treatment.

Social anxiety disorder severity scales such as the Liebowitz Social Anxiety Symptom Scale (Appendix A) and measures of disability such as the Sheehan Disability Scale (Appendix B) have been developed to assess a patient's degree of impairment (see Appendices C and D for additional diagnostic tools/severity scales for social anxiety disorder). These scales provide a good indication of what assessments are necessary to appraise the severity of symptoms.

Introducing the issue of treatment

Many sufferers of social anxiety disorder will never have heard of the condition. They may think of their symptoms as extreme shyness or as some unfortunate trait of personality and therefore need to be convinced that a long-term treatment plan can be of help.

Spending some time to explain the rationale for pharmacotherapy can therefore greatly improve patient compliance.

There are five complimentary strategies for presenting the issue of medication to a patient:

- Emphasize that social anxiety disorder is a well-documented medical condition that has been shown in many studies to respond well to appropriate treatment.

- Explain that the phobic avoidance is driven by anxiety. Medication can directly alleviate this anxiety.

- In generalized social anxiety disorder explain that excessive vulnerability to rejection or criticism can be specifically modified by certain pharmacotherapeutic regimens.

- Explain that drug treatment is not addictive or habit-forming and does not cause withdrawal symptoms when stopped.

- Establish a treatment contract with the patient.

The treatment contract

A formal contract addressing the issue of treatment can be a valuable aid to compliance. The contract should

- Reframe the patient's symptoms as social anxiety disorder

- Emphasize that social anxiety disorder is a recognized medical condition that responds well to treatment

- Negotiate treatment

- List problems and priorities

- Set a realistic time scale for improvement

- Agree to review the medication regularly

How long to treat

It is important to emphasize to the patient that social anxiety disorder is a chronic condition that is likely to require long-term management.

Even when treatment is maintained for 6 months, there is a relapse rate of about 20% to 50% once the medication is withdrawn.

EVALUATING CLINICAL RESPONSE

The outcome of a pharmacologic intervention may be evaluated by looking for meaningful improvement in the following areas:

- Anxiety experienced during a social encounter or performance event and possibly quality of performance and social interaction
- Anxiety experienced in anticipation of the feared situation (anticipatory anxiety)
- Avoidance of social encounters or obligations, relationship opportunities, or performance
- Comorbidity related to the social anxiety disorder, such as secondary depression, demoralization, or alcohol abuse
- Overall functional impairment due to the social anxiety disorder

Adapted from Heimberg RG, et al.: Social Phobia Diagnosis, Assessment and Treatment London: The Guilford Press; 1995.

Drug therapy should therefore be withdrawn gradually, with periodic attempts to lower the dose.

Strategy for nonresponders

Pharmacotherapy should be initiated with the most effective and safest options available. After a realistic period of treatment (1 to 2 months) the clinical response should be evaluated (*see* table). If the patient remains significantly impaired, the physician may consider increasing to the maximum effective dose or using another class of medication. The addition of psychologic therapies to the drug regimen may also be considered.

Selection of Medication

The pharmacologic agents generally found to be most effective against social anxiety disorder are those that effect serotonin. These include selective serotonin reuptake inhibitors (SSRIs) and MAOIs. The benzodiazepine drug, clonazepam, which also has serotonergic properties, is effective in social anxiety disorder. Beta-blockers may be sometimes effective on limited autonomic symptoms in performance settings; the tricyclic drug imipramine appears to be ineffective, and buspirone may have some effects at higher doses.

SSRIs

Recent studies have indicated that the SSRI paroxetine is effective in double-blind, placebo-controlled trials. Currently the data are unpublished but are based on substantial sample sizes. Two smaller open-label trials have attested to the benefits of paroxetine. In a trial by Stein *et al.* (1996), 77% of subjects completing 11 weeks of treatment were judged to be responders, and symptoms were reduced on the Brief Social Phobia Scale (BSPS) from 34.1 down to 17.5. Paroxetine responders were then randomized to remain on drug for an additional 12 weeks or receive placebo double-blind. Relapse rates were 12.5% for those remaining on drug, versus 62.5% for those switched to placebo. This study suggests that paroxetine produces a positive acute effect, and that the relapse rate after discontinuing treatment at 3 months is substantial.

In a second study of paroxetine, Mancini and Van Ameringen found an 83% response rate among 18 patients who receive paroxetine at 12 weeks. Mean doses of paroxetine in the two studies were 47.9 and 36.1 mg per day, respectively.

Open-label studies of fluoxetine have suggested that there is benefit for the drug, and that its clinical effects may be related to brain levels of fluoxetine as measured by magnetic resonance spectroscopy (Miner *et al.*; 1995). One small double-blind placebo-controlled crossover trial has shown that sertraline exceeds placebo with respect to therapeutic outcome (Katzelnick *et al.*, 1994). Fluvoxamine has been studied in two double-blind trials (van Vliet *et al.*, 1994 and Stein *et al.*, unpublished), both studies indicating positive effects for the drug relative to placebo. The second study was conducted in primarily generalized social anxiety disorder patients, who for the most part seem to form the great bulk of clinical trial samples.

MAOIs

The MAOI phenelzine has been shown to have an acute benefit in 60% to 75% of treated patients, with significant clinical improvement seen after 8 to 12 weeks of therapy. Phenelzine remains effective with continued administration, although there is a substantial rate of relapse once the therapy is withdrawn.

One potential problem with phenelzine therapy is persuading patients to comply with the therapy.

A number of problematic side effects can lead to a large proportion of patients withdrawing from the treatment program before receiving the full benefits of therapy. These side effects include hypertensive crisis (if dietary restrictions on tyramine intake are not followed), insomnia, sexual dysfunction, postural hypertension, and weight gain.

Other irreversible MAOIs besides phenelzine have been studied, although there is an absence of data from controlled trials. Two open trials of tranylcypromine both suggested a therapeutic effect.

Benzodiazepines

Benzodiazepines do not enjoy a reputation for being useful in social anxiety disorder.

The possible exception is clonazepam, which also has serotonergic effects. One placebo-controlled trial that followed 75 patients receiving either clonazepam or placebo for 10 weeks found that 78% of patients on the benzodiazepine responded to therapy compared with just 20% on placebo.

There are, however, drawbacks to treating social anxiety disorder with benzodiazepines, not least of which is the danger of physical dependency in patients on long-term therapy. The link between social anxiety disorder and alcohol abuse also suggests that benzodiazepines may not be the treatment of choice for many sufferers. One double-blind discontinuation study of clonazepam has shown that it can be safely withdrawn, if done slowly, after 6 months of treatment, with a small risk of increased relapse and some clinical worsening.

Beta-blockers

There is little evidence to suggest that beta-blockers have any beneficial effect on the underlying disease in social anxiety disorder.

However, they can be useful when taken acutely to combat the tremor, palpitations, and tachycardia often experienced by social anxiety disorder sufferers in specific performance situations.

For this reason many social anxiety disorder patients use medications such as propranolol on an as-needed basis.

Other agents
Open studies have suggested a number of other agents may be of use in combating social anxiety disorder such as the non-benzodiazepine anxiolytic buspirone previously mentioned.

Recent magnetic resonance studies in social anxiety disorder
Three magnetic resonance spectroscopy studies have been conducted in social anxiety disorder by Davidson and colleagues. In the first two reports, increases were noted in brain choline relative to *N*-acetyl-aspartate. In the second study, *myo*-inositol was also measured and found to be present in higher quantities relative to *N*-acetyl-aspartate. The relevance of these findings could relate to the proxy role served by choline and *myo*-inositol as downstream markers of altered serotonin or dopamine activity or receptor sensitivity in social anxiety disorder.

In the third study, brain levels of fluoxetine were found to correlate with the effect of that drug in social anxiety disorder in a small sample of subjects.

Comorbidity
One of the major problems in treating social anxiety disorder is the extremely high prevalence of comorbid conditions.

As a general rule it is preferable to treat with a single agent that is known to be efficacious for each disorder separately. If one disorder is clearly believed to be secondary then therapy may focus on the primary condition. Copharmacy, using compatible agents effective for individual disorders may be necessary.

When social anxiety disorder appears together with depression, treatment should involve antidepressants known to be effective against both disorders, such as SSRIs and MAOIs.

SSRIs are the first-line treatment for social anxiety disorder. However, patients with social anxiety disorder comorbid with obsessive-compulsive disorder were recently found to respond less well to SSRIs than to MAOIs.

When treating social anxiety disorder patients with concomitant panic disorder or any history of unexpected panic symptoms, SSRIs need to be started at very low doses to avoid exacerbation of the panic symptoms.

Due to the risk of dependency, benzodiazepine therapy should be employed with caution.

Psychologic Treatment of Social Anxiety Disorder

The rationale for psychologic treatment is to encourage sufferers to confront negative beliefs—such as thinking failure is inevitable in social situations—thought to be at the root of their social anxiety disorder.

Cognitive therapies in the management of social anxiety disorder produce positive results, although a number of caveats must be added to their conclusions. Most of the studies were very small and had insufficient power to test adequately the therapy's efficacy. There is also a major difficulty in developing truly neutral controls or behavioral treatments. A more recent larger study by Heimberg and Liebowitz, as yet unpublished, suggests promising benefit.

Because one of the main goals of cognitive therapy is to encourage patients to confront their anxieties, group therapy sessions are particularly appropriate to the treatment of social anxiety disorder. Psychologic techniques may be used as an adjuvant or alternative to pharmacologic therapy.

Summary

Social anxiety disorder responds well to treatment.

Early intervention may help prevent severe impairment, the development of harmful coping strategies, and the onset of comorbid conditions such as major depression and alcoholism.

Treatment should be initiated in cases in which symptoms or avoidance behavior are associated with significant psychosocial impairment.

Explaining the rationale for pharmacotherapy and that the treatment is likely to be needed for some time may help patient compliance.

The pharmacologic agents found to be most effective in social anxiety disorder are SSRIs and MAOIs. Because the safety profiles of the SSRIs are better than those of the MAOIs, SSRIs should be considered first-line treatment. Other agents used in the treatment of social anxiety disorder include benzodiazepines and beta-blockers.

Psychologic therapy used either in isolation or in combination with drug therapy may also be a useful treatment approach.

APPENDIX A: LIEBOWITZ SOCIAL ANXIETY SYMPTOM SCALE

Rate all items using the past week, including today, as the frame of reference. If any situation did not occur in the past week, rate according to how the patient says he/she would have reacted if confronted by the situation. For each situation rate both the degree of fear or anxiety that was or would have been experienced and the frequency with which the patient avoided or would have avoided the situation.

		Fear or Anxiety 1 = None 2 = Mild 3 = Moderate 4 = Severe	Avoidance 1 = Never (0%) 2 = Occasionally (1%–33%) 3 = Often (34%–67%) 4 = Usually (68%–100%)
1. Using a telephone in public	P	[ ]	[ ]
2. Participating in a small group activity	P	[ ]	[ ]
3. Eating in public	P	[ ]	[ ]
4. Drinking in public	P	[ ]	[ ]
5. Talking to someone in authority	S	[ ]	[ ]
6. Acting, performing, or speaking in front of an audience	P	[ ]	[ ]
7. Going to a party	S	[ ]	[ ]
8. Working while being observed	P	[ ]	[ ]
9. Writing while being observed	P	[ ]	[ ]
10. Telephoning someone you don't know very well	S	[ ]	[ ]

11.	Talking face to face with someone you don't know very well	S	[ ] [ ]
12.	Meeting strangers	S	[ ] [ ]
13.	Urinating in a public bathroom	P	[ ] [ ]
14.	Entering a room when others are already seated	P	[ ] [ ]
15.	Being the center of attention	S	[ ] [ ]
16.	Speaking up at a meeting without advance preparation	P	[ ] [ ]
17.	Taking a test of your ability, skill, or knowledge	P	[ ] [ ]
18.	Expressing disagreement or disapproval to someone you don't know very well	S	[ ] [ ]
19.	Looking "straight in the eyes" of someone you don't know very well	S	[ ] [ ]
20.	Giving a prepared oral report to a group	P	[ ] [ ]
21.	Trying to make someone's acquaintance for the purpose of a romantic/sexual relationship (a pick-up)	P	[ ] [ ]
22.	Returning goods or merchandise to a store to obtain a refund	S	[ ] [ ]
23.	Giving a party	S	[ ] [ ]
24.	Resisting a high-pressure sales person	S	[ ] [ ]

APPENDIX B: SHEEHAN DISABILITIES SCALE

On a scale of 0 to 10, as shown on the diagram below, enter the number that best describes the amount of your disability or impairment, at this time, in each of the following areas: Work, Social Life and Activities, and Family Life and Home Responsibilities.

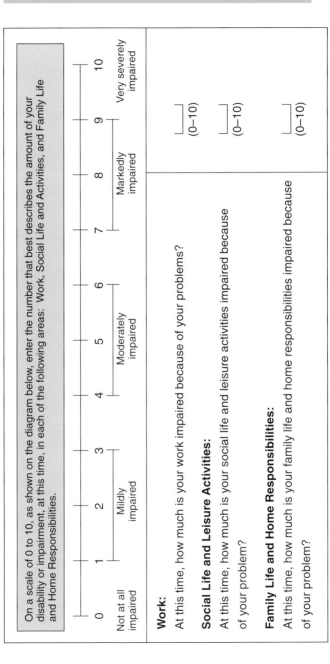

0	1	2	3	4	5	6	7	8	9	10
Not at all impaired		Mildly impaired			Moderately impaired			Markedly impaired		Very severely impaired

Work:

At this time, how much is your work impaired because of your problems?

[ ] (0–10)

Social Life and Leisure Activities:

At this time, how much is your social life and leisure activities impaired because of your problem?

[ ] (0–10)

Family Life and Home Responsibilities:

At this time, how much is your family life and home responsibilities impaired because of your problem?

[ ] (0–10)

■ APPENDIX C: SOCIAL PHOBIA INVENTORY

Please check how the following problems have bothered you during the past week. Mark only one box for each problem and be sure to answer all items.

	Not at all	A little bit	Somewhat	Very much	Extremely
1. I am afraid of people in authority.	☐	☐	☐	☐	☐
2. I am bothered by blushing in front of people.	☐	☐	☐	☐	☐
3. Parties and social events scare me.	☐	☐	☐	☐	☐
4. I avoid talking to people I don't know.	☐	☐	☐	☐	☐
5. Being criticized scares me a lot.	☐	☐	☐	☐	☐
6. Fear of embarrassment causes me to avoid doing things or speaking to people.	☐	☐	☐	☐	☐
7. Sweating in front of people causes me distress.	☐	☐	☐	☐	☐
8. I avoid going to parties.	☐	☐	☐	☐	☐
9. I avoid activities in which I am the center of attention.	☐	☐	☐	☐	☐

☐	☐	☐	☐	☐	☐	☐	☐
☐	☐	☐	☐	☐	☐	☐	☐
☐	☐	☐	☐	☐	☐	☐	☐
☐	☐	☐	☐	☐	☐	☐	☐

10. Talking to strangers scares me.

11. I avoid having to give speeches.

12. I would do anything to avoid being criticized.

13. Heart palpitations bother me when I am around people.

14. I am afraid of doing things when people might be watching.

15. Being embarrassed or looking stupid are among my worst fears.

16. I avoid speaking to anyone in authority.

17. Trembling or shaking in front of others is distressing to me.

Courtesy of JRT Davidson, MD.

APPENDIX D: BRIEF SOCIAL PHOBIA SCALE

Instructions

The clinician will rate the time period covering the previous week. If a patient has not been exposed to the feared situation in the past week, the clinician should rate the fear, avoidance, and physiologic symptoms according to how the patient would feel now if faced with each situation.

Part I (fear/avoidance)

How much do you fear and avoid the following situations? The clinician will give separate ratings for fear and avoidance by recording in each box below a score corresponding with the following clinical anchor points.

	Fear	Avoidance
1. Speaking in public or in front of others	☐	☐
2. Talking to people in authority	☐	☐
3. Talking to strangers	☐	☐
4. Being embarrassed or humiliated	☐	☐
5. Being criticized	☐	☐
6. Social gatherings	☐	☐
7. Doing something while being watched (this does not include speaking)	☐	☐

Clinical anchor points

Fear:

0 = None
1 = Mild—Infrequent and/or not distressing
2 = Moderate—Frequent and/or some distress
3 = Severe—Constant, dominating a person's life and/or clearly distressing
4 = Extreme—Incapacitating and/or very painfully distressing

Avoidance:

0 = Never (0%)
1 = Rare (1%–33%)
2 = Sometimes (34%–66%)
3 = Frequent (67%–99%)
4 = Always (100%)

Part II (physiologic)

When you are in a situation that involves contact with other people, or when you are thinking about such a situation, do you experience the following symptoms? Record in each box below a score corresponding with the following clinical anchor points.

Physiologic

1. Blushing ☐

2. Palpitations ☐

3. Trembling or shaking ☐

4. Sweating ☐

Clinical anchor points

Physiologic:
0=None
1=Mild—Infrequent and/or not distressing
2=Moderate—Frequent and/or some distress
3=Severe—Constant, dominating a person's life and/or clearly distressing
4=Extreme—Incapacitating and/or very painfully distressing

Total scores

Part I	Fear items 1–7	Total____	(F)
	Avoidance items 1–7	Total____	(A)
Part II	Physiologic items 1–4	Total____	(P)
(F+A+P)		**Total____**	

■ REFERENCES

American Psychiatric Association: *Diagnostic and Statistical Manual of Mental Disorders*, edn 4. American Psychiatric Association: Washington DC; 1994.

American Psychiatric Association: *Diagnostic and Statistical Manual of Mental Disorders*, edn 3. American Psychiatric Association: Washington DC; 1987.

Amies PL, *et al.*: Social phobia: a comparative clinical study. *Br J Psychiatry* 1983, 142:174–179.

Bisserbe JC, *et al.*: Moclobemide in social phobia: a pilot open study. *Clin Neuropharmacol* 1994, 17(suppl 1):S88–S94.

Black B, *et al.*: Fluoxetine for the treatment of social phobia. *J Clin Psychopharmacol* 1992, 12:293–295.

Bowen RC, *et al.*: Alcoholism, anxiety disorders, and agoraphobia. *Alcohol Clin Exp Res* 1984, 8:48–50.

Brewerton TD, *et al.*: Eating disorders and social phobia [letter]. *Arch Gen Psychiatry* 1993, 50:70.

Carrasco JL, *et al.*: Treatment outcome of obsessive compulsive disorder with comorbid social phobia. *J Clin Psychiatry* 1992, 53:387–391.

Chambless DL, *et al.*: *J Anxiety Disord* 1987, 1:29–40.

Clark DB, *et al.*: The assessment and treatment of performance anxiety in musicians. *Am J Psychiatry* 1991, 148:598–605.

Cox BJ, *et al.*: Suicidal ideation and suicide attempts in panic disorder and social phobia. *Am J Psychiatry* l994, 151:882–887.

Davidson JR, *et al.*: Treatment of social phobia with clonazepam and placebo. *J Clin Psychopharmacol* 1993, 13:423–428.

Davidson JR, *et al.*: The epidemiology of social phobia: findings from the Duke Epidemiological Catchment Area Study. *Psychol Med* 1993, 23:709–718.

Davidson JR, *et al.*: Magnetic resonance spectroscopy in social phobia: preliminary findings. *J Clin Psychiatry* 1993, 54(suppl):19–25.

Degonda M, Angst J: The Zurich study: XX: social phobia and agoraphobia. *Eur Arch Psychiatry Clin Neurosci* 1993, 243:95–102.

Den Boer JA, *et al.*: *Prog Neuropsychopharmacol Biol Psychiatry*1994, 18:634–636.

DeRuiter C, *et al.*: *J Anxiety Disord*1989, 3:57–68.

Eaton WW, *et al.*: *Psychiatric Disorders in America: The Epidemiological Catchment Area Study.* New York: The Free Press; 1991:155–179.

Emmanuel NP, *et al.*: Treatment of social phobia with bupropion. *J Clin Psychopharmacol* 1991, 11:276–277.

Falloon IR, *et al.*: The treatment of social phobia: real-life rehearsal with nonprofessional therapists. *J Nerv Ment Dis* 1981, 169:180–184.

Gelernter CS, *et al.*: Cognitive-behavioral and pharmacological treatments of social phobia: a controlled study. *Arch Gen Psychiatry* 1991, 48:938–945.

Gelernter CS, *et al.*: An examination of syndromal validity and diagnostic subtypes in social phobia and panic disorder. *J Clin Psychiatry* 1992, 53:23–27.

Goldstein S: Treatment of social phobia with clonidine. *Biol Psychiatry* 1987, 22:369–372.

Gorman OM, *et al.*: Treatment of social phobia with atenolol. *J Clin Psychopharmacol* 1985, 5:298–301.

Heimberg RG, *et al.*: *J Anxiety Disord* 1993, 7:249–269.

Heimberg RG, *et al.*: *Social Phobia Diagnosis, Assessment and Treatment.* London: The Guilford Press; 1995.

Horwath E, *et al.*: Agoraphobia without panic: clinical reappraisal of an epidemiologic finding. *Am J Psychiatry* 1993, 150:1496–1501.

International Multicentre Study Group. Presented by Buller R at ECMP, Jerusalem, 1994.

Kendler KS, *et al.*: The genetic epidemiology of phobias in women: the interrelationship of agoraphobia, social phobia, situational phobia, and simple phobia. *Arch Gen Psychiatry* 1992, 49:273–281.

Kessler RC, *et al.*: Lifetime and 12-month prevalence of DSM-III-R psychiatric disorders in the United States: results from the National Comorbidity Survey. *Arch Gen Psychiatry* 1994, 51:8–19.

Kushner MG, *et al.*: The relation between alcohol problems and the anxiety disorders. *Am J Psychiatry* 1990, 147:685–695.

Lepine J-P, *et al.*: *International Journal of Methods in Psychiatric Research* 1993, 3:67–77.

Liebowitz MR, *et al.*: Social phobia: review of a neglected anxiety disorder. *Arch Gen Psychiatry* 1985, 42:729–736.

Liebowitz MR, *et al.*: Phenelzine vs atenolol in social phobia: a placebo-controlled comparison. *Arch Gen Psychiatry* 1992, 49:290–300.

Lydiard RB, *et al.*: Alprazolam in the treatment of social phobia. *J Clin Psychiatry* 1988, 49:17–19.

Marshall JR: The diagnosis and treatment of social phobia and alcohol abuse. *Bull Menninger Clin* 1994, 58(suppl A):A58–A66.

Merikangas KR: *Eur Arch Psychiatry Clin Neurosci* 1995, 294:207–303.

Merikangas KR, Angst J: *Eur Neuropsychopharmacol* 1993, 3:188–189.

Miner CM, *et al.*: Brain fluoxetine measurements using fluorine magnetic resonance spectroscopy in patients with social phobia. *Biol Psychiatry* 1995, 38:696–698.

Mullaney JA, *et al.*: Alcohol dependence and phobias: clinical description and relevance. *Br J Psychiatry* 1979, 135:565–573.

Munjack DJ, *et al*.: *J Anxiety Disord* 1991, 5:87–98.

Oest L-G: Age of onset in different phobias. *J Abnorm Psychol* 1987, 96:223–229.

Reich JH, *et al*.: Alprazolam treatment of avoidant personality traits in social phobic patients. *J Clin Psychiatry* 1989, 50:91–95.

Reich JH, *et al*.: *J Nerv Ment Dis* 1994, 182:297–301.

Reiter SR, *et al*.: Clonazepam for the treatment of social phobia. *J Clin Psychiatry* 1990, 51:470–472.

Ross J: Social phobia: the Anxiety Disorders Associated of America helps raise the veil of ignorance. *J Clin Psychiatry* 1991, 52(suppl 11):43–47.

Ross J: Social phobia: the consumer's perspective. *J Clin Psychiatry* 1993, 54 (suppl):5–9.

Schneier FR, *et al*.: *J Anxiety Disord* 1989, 3:15–23.

Schneier FR, *et al*.: Social phobia: comorbidity and morbidity in an epidemiologic sample. *Arch Gen Psychiatry* 1992, 49:282–288.

Schneier FR, *et al*.: Fluoxetine in social phobia. *J Clin Psychopharmacol* 1992, 12:62–64.

Schneier FR, *et al*.: Buspirone in social phobia. *J Clin Psychopharmacol* 1993, 13:251–256.

Schwalberg MD, *et al*.: Comparison of bulimics, obese binge eaters, social phobics, and individuals with panic disorder on comorbidity across DSM-III-R anxiety disorders. *J Abnorm Psychol* 1992, 101:675–681.

Smail P, *et al*.: Alcohol dependence and phobic anxiety states. *Br J Psychiatry* 1984, 144:53–57.

Solyom L, *et al*.: Delineating social phobia. *Br J Psychiatry* 1986, 149:464–470.

Stein DJ, *et al*.: Setting diagnostic thresholds for social phobia: considerations from a community survey of social anxiety. *Am J Psychiatry* 1994, 151:408–412.

Sternbach H: Fluoxetine treatment of social phobia. *J Clin Psychopharmacol* 1990, 10:230–231.

Stravynski A, *et al*.: Clinical phobias and avoidant personality disorder among alcoholics admitted to an alcoholism rehabilitation setting. *Can J Psychiatry* 1986, 31:714–719.

Swinson RP, *et al*.: Use of medical services and treatment for panic disorder with agoraphobia and for social phobia. *Can Med Assoc J* 1992, 147:878–883.

Thyer BA, *et al*.: Alcohol abuse among clinically anxious patients. *Behav Res Ther* 1986, 24:357–359.

Tupler LA, *et al*.: A repeat proton magnetic resonance spectroscopy study in social phobia. *Biol Psychiatry* 1997, 42:419–424.

Turner SM, Beidel DC: *Clin Psychol Rev* 1989, 9:3–18.

Turner SM, *et al.*: Social phobia: a comparison of behavior therapy and atenolol. *J Consult Clin Psychol* 1994, 62:350–358.

US Multicentre Study Group. Presented by Buller R at ECMP, Jerusalem, 1994.

Van Ameringen M, *et al.*: Relationship of social phobia with other psychiatric illness. *J Affect Disord* 1991, 21:93–99.

Van Ameringen M, *et al.*: Fluoxetine efficacy in social phobia. *J Clin Psychiatry* 1993, 54:27–32.

Versiani M, *et al.*: Tranylcypromine in social phobia. *J Clin Psychopharmacol* 1988, 8:279–283.

Versiani M, *et al.*: *Journal Brasileiro de Psiquiatria* 1989, 38:251–263.

Versiani M, *et al.*: Pharmacotherapy of social phobia: a controlled study with moclobemide and phenelzine. *Br J Psychiatry* 1992, 161:353–360.

van Vliet IM, *et al.*: Psychopharmacological treatment of social phobia: clinical and biochemical effects of brofaromine, a selective MAO-A inhibitor. *Eur Neuropsychopharmacol* 1992, 2:21–29.

Wacker HR, *et al.*: *International Journal of Methods in Psychiatric Research* 1992, 2:91–100.

World Health Organization: *International Classification of Diseases*, 10th revision: Chapter V, Mental and Behavioural Disorders (ICD-10). WHO: Geneva; 1990.

■ INDEX